I0421658

Natural Deodorant:

Easy Recipes For Homemade and Extremely Effective Body Deodorants

Disclamer: All photos used in this book, including the cover photo were made available under a Attribution-NonCommercial-ShareAlike 2.0 Generic and sourced from Flickr

Table of Content:

Introduction

Modern girls find it difficult to imagine the morning without the use of the favorite deodorant. But how often do we consider the fact that the harm from this product is bigger than benefit? The debate about the safety of antiperspirants has been going on almost since they appeared on the shelves of pharmacies. The detrimental effect of these cosmetics is due to the presence of aluminum and zinc.

Getting on the skin, antiperspirant forms a special film. Its task is to block the sweat glands, and, therefore, to prevent the occurrence of an unpleasant odor. But not everything is so simple. Sweating is a natural property of the human body. With its help, toxic substances are removed and the body temperature is maintained. Simply put, the use of antiperspirant interferes with natural cleansing.

If you ask doctors, you will suddenly know the shocking truth. Particularly, the use of antiperspirants is one of the causes of breast cancer. This is due to the action of parabens - preservatives, commonly used in the cosmetic industry.

The carcinogenicity of these substances is still questionable, but many women are already switching to natural self-care products. What is to replace the antiperspirant from the store? The best option is a tool made with your own hands.

Which benefits does home-made deodorant have?

Firstly, they do not contain any health risks. Consider the difference between antiperspirant and deodorant. Many believe that this is the same thing but there are significant differences in the operation of these means. For instance, the antiperspirant clogs the glands and blocks sweating

Deodorant, in turn, destroys microorganisms that live in the ducts of sweat glands and cause an unpleasant smell. At the same time the process of sweating is preserved, and harmful substances do not linger in the body. Deodorants are difficult to find in stores, but can be made from scrap materials.

As well, such recipes of homemade deodorants are approved by several generations. The beneficial properties of soda, citrus essential oils and cocoa were successfully used long before the mass production of cosmetics.

Finally, in contrast to the "biting" prices of cosmetics of famous brands, the cost of the components of home deodorant will delight you. Ingredients for such a tool can be found in the kitchen or bought at a nearby supermarket.

Chapter 1 – Why people all over the world opt for natural deodorants

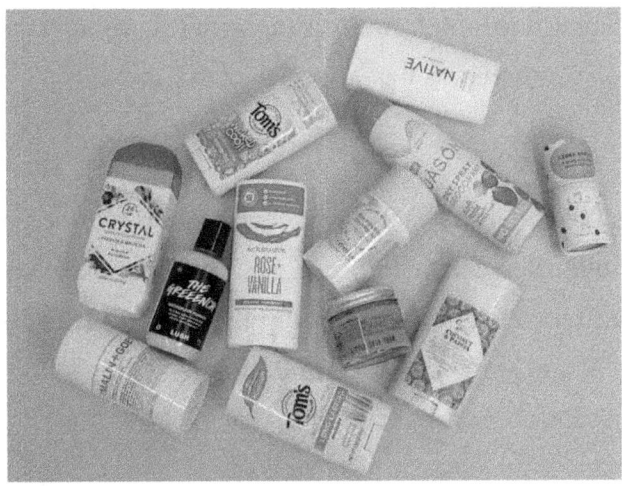

Today more and more people all around the world are making their choice in favor of natural deodorants. Not only do they reject from the chemical analogues but also dedicate their time to creation of deodorants on their own.

Sweating is a natural process that allows the body to maintain a constant temperature, and it helps us we feel quite comfortable. But if a person sweats intensely, it affects the quality of his life badly. Such a situation is getting abnormal, that's why people can speak about hyperhidrosis, mean, excessive sweating.

The same applies to the strong smell of sweat, a condition called bromidrosis. Everyone tries to cope with this problem in different ways, but often the chosen means are ineffective and sometimes even harmful. In most cases, excessive sweating is just a feature of the body.

If you are actively sweating from adolescence or at least 25 years old, then this is the case. An unpleasant odor occurs due to the fact that bacteria recycle compounds contained in sweat and skin, and as a result, bad-smelling substances such as ammonia are formed.

It can be especially noticeable among people with too much sweat - the bacteria in these favorable conditions become larger and the scale of production of odorous substances increases. That is, bromidrosis and hyperhidrosis are often related phenomena.

Although sometimes it may be that a person has too many specific sweat glands (apocrine), which secrete not a liquid, but a fatty substance (mostly it happens when a person is nervous). Because of that, smell appears.

If excessive sweating appears after the person is over 25 years old, it can be the cause of some disease or medication, especially if a person is sweating at night or suddenly lost weight. There is a great deal of diseases and conditions leading to hyperhidrosis, from menopause to tuberculosis.

Therefore, it is better not to deal with the symptoms, but go to the doctor who will find the cause. There is absolutely no need to hesitate whether it is worth visiting a specialist if there is dizziness, chest pain or nausea. There are also quite a lot of medications for which a person begins to sweat more intensively (among them, for example, nitroglycerin and some antidepressants), but you shouldn't stop them without a doctor.

An unpleasant smell of sweat from the whole body, and not from the legs or armpits, can also be a sign of the disease, but usually in this case there are other severe symptoms. More often the case is in the diet - garlic, onion, curry and alcohol can affect the smell of sweat. Antiperspirants and deodorants are the next things a doctor will recommend after basic hygiene practices.

Deodorants should mask the smell of sweat, that is, one smell should interrupt the other. They also often contain alcohol, which results in the formation of an acidic environment on the skin that is uncomfortable for bacteria. The effectiveness of this approach is not very large, and deodorants can save only in the easiest cases.

Antiperspirants work because aluminum salts (usually aluminum chloride, also aluminum chloride hexahydrate) clog pores from which sweat comes out. Theoretically, even the most common antiperspirants (with a low concentration of aluminum salts) can cause swelling and irritation of the skin, but in practice this is quite rare.

Do not be afraid of the fact that over time there will be addiction to antiperspirants and they will have to be applied more often. Antiperspirants need to be used correctly. Ordinary antiperspirants are recommended to be applied after a shower on dry skin. However, right after this, you should not sweat for the remedy to work. Therefore, the American Academy of Dermatology generally advises the use of antiperspirants before bedtime.

Antiperspirants, in which the concentration of aluminum chloride is above 6%, are also recommended to be applied to clean, dry skin at bedtime. Because of numerous problems connected to the deodorants and antiperspirants which we have bought in the shops, nowadays more and more people tend to make this product at home.

We will tell you how to do it with the least efforts.

Chapter 2 – The most harmful ingredients which you never need in deodorants

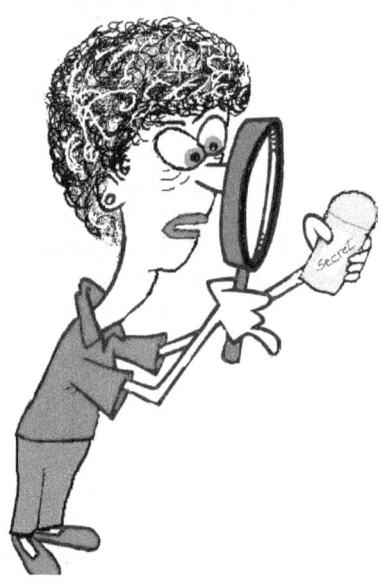

Why do you need a substitute for deodorant? Now the market proposes a lot of deodorants of different shapes, smell and composition. However, they also contain hazardous substances, such as aluminum. We use deodorant every day, rubbing it into the skin. In such a way aluminum penetrates the body, causing hormonal disruptions, premature aging, Alzheimer's disease and even cancer. Sometimes it may not contain aluminum, but it is often replaced by other chemicals.

Doctors have proven that sweat is the usual moisture that our glands secrete, and it does not smell. The smell comes from bacteria that are actively developing in a humid environment, and it may depend on gender, diet, drugs, and other factors. Vegetarians claim that the rejection of animal food helps to get rid of the unpleasant smell of sweat.

If you care about your health but don't believe how important natural deodorants are, pay attention to the chemical components in your product. It can be aluminum as it clogs the sweat glands, after which swelling may occur.

The next harmful component is paraben used as preservatives. This substance causes allergies, in severe cases, asphyxiation. Next, triclosan is considered as the most dangerous "killer" of bacteria. Along with the bacteria that cause smell, it destroys the beneficial protective microflora of the skin.

Perhaps, you have never heard about it, but triclosan is banned for use in cosmetics in America and Europe. Then, it comes down to deodorants. Synthetic fragrances give deodorants a pleasant smell. However, it quickly disappears, and the perfumes have time to harm health.

After that, propylene glycol is the substance is antibacterial, but causes problems with the liver and kidneys. In the United States and Europe, its use is prohibited. Finally, alcohol that has a bactericidal effect may cause dryness and irritation.

Indeed, only because of our laziness and lack of desire to create a new product hand-made, we push ourselves in the depth of harmful elements which poison our bodies inside.

So, which things are necessary for beautiful look, amazing smell, and good health condition?

Chapter 3 – The best components to include in natural deodorants

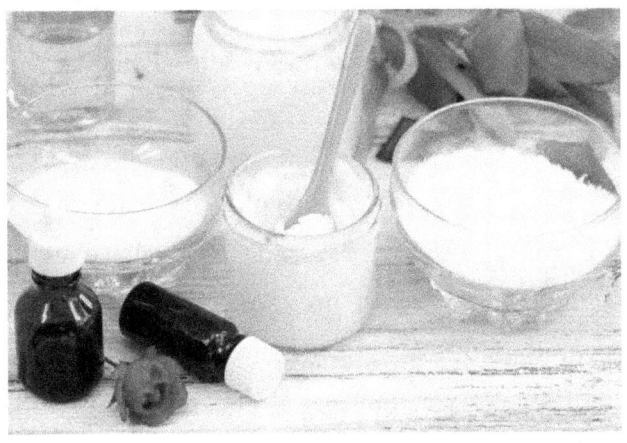

Natural deodorants substitutes contain natural ingredients: *essential oils, coconut oil, natural starch, and alum stone.*The problem of unpleasant smell was tried to be solved even before the invention of deodorants. By the way, in clothes from natural fabrics it is less noticeable.

Try using a natural substitute for deodorants, and you will see the result immediately! Not only will you like the smell, but also you are about to feel healthier. Soda is the most popular "wrestler" with a smell. Soda will not stop sweating, but at the same time, won't allow bacteria to multiply.

Soda can be used in different forms; particularly, it might be dry as a powder. Then, it is likely to bring a perfect solution in warm water for rinsing or a mixture with starch, to reduce the "moisture". In such a powder for the smell, you can add a few drops of essential oils.

Regular baking soda can be diluted in water and wiped with an armpit cotton pad. It does not relieve sweat, but there is no smell. On very hot days, the procedure should be repeated. However, one factor should be taken in consideration. If you have very sensitive skin, soda can overdry it. Thus, everything is good when it is measured.

In case you are into different sophisticated tastes, you choice has to turn next to essential oils. They are extremely pleasant, and have smoothing and healing effect on the skin and total emotional state.

Oil of lavender, fir, pine, tea tree, geranium, wormwood, rosemary, fennel, clove, orange tree, eucalyptus, bergamot, cedar and thyme have antiseptic properties.It is a good idea to apply oil to your finger and rub into areas where there is an unpleasant smell.

Once you are fond of fresh fruits or feel thirsty during the hot days, you might rub into the skin the sap of lemon or water-based apple cider vinegar. The aim of this substance changes the acidity of the skin and causes a deodorizing effect.

As well, coconut oil can be the basis of natural deodorant. If you want to make it natural, add *to 5 teaspoons of coconut oil 1/4 cup soda, 1/4 cup starch and essential oils.* First mix the dry ingredients (starch and soda), and then coconut oil. If the oil is too thick, heat it in a microwave or in a water bath. You can also add wax.

The mixture is placed in a jar or in a package from under the deodorant and use as an ordinary deodorant. Keep better in the refrigerator.

Herbs are also necessary. Infusions of calamus, willow bark, wormwood, thyme, chamomile, coriander are made in cold water, and not boiled. If you have desire to use oak bark, you are highly likely to prepare a decoction. It might be done in the following way: take 1 tablespoon of crushed bark in a glass of water.

Afterwards, wet the cotton pad in the broth and wipe the body. As a substitute for deodorant, burnt alum (aluminum potassium alum) is widely used, but it is aluminum salts, which adversely affects the brain, causes allergies, and damages the immune system.

The most convenient option is a mixture based on oils. Ingredients (essential oils, soda, starch, beeswax) are easy to buy and cook very simply. This deodorant can use a year. After the deodorant has been applied, wait 5 minutes so that there are no marks on the clothes.

Chapter 4 – How to create deodorants from coconut and vanilla?

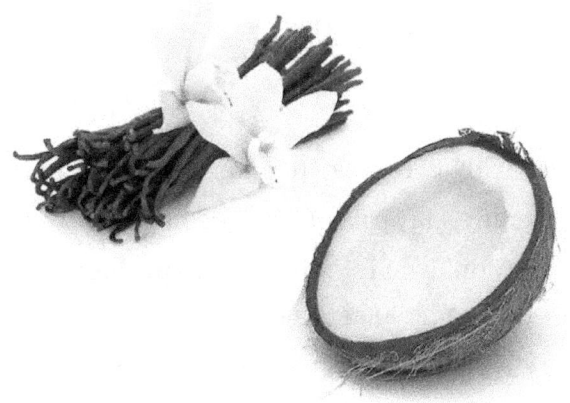

Natural deodorant for the body does not clog pores, does not contain aluminum, lead, parabens. Unfortunately, all these harmful substances are contained in industrial deodorants. They have a peculiarity to accumulate in the body, moreover, it is believed that they can cause breast cancer.

In the modern rhythm of life, many people cannot survive without deodorant, and continue to consciously poison themselves with chemistry to disguise an undesirable smell, this is not the way out.

So, you might try to make your own hands a simple, natural and safe for health deodorant. Its production will take not so much time, and all the ingredients that you need, you can easily find on the shelves of shops, pharmacies or on the Internet.

Let's start with two most popular smells of the modern aroma therapy, in particular, coconut oil and vanilla. Firstly, why don't you try **solid natural deodorant with coconut oil**! For that, you need 50 grams of soda. Actually, have you ever heard that baking soda itself is a natural deodorizer?

The next ingredient is 50 grams of corn starch which absorbs, protects and dries the skin. Tea tree essential oil is necessary in the amount of 8-10 drops. However, if desired, you can increase or decrease the amount of essential oil or replace it with another.

Concerning the coconut oil, 2-3 tablespoons will be enough. It is necessary because of ability to soften and moisturize the skin. It is quickly absorbed, and does not leave a fat mark. Also, it serves to impart hardness to deodorant.

When everything is ready, you should follow the next steps:

1. Mix soda with corn starch, add essential oil of tea tree.

2. Next, add coconut oil, which can be pre-melted in a water bath to better mix the ingredients.

3. Put the mixture in the tube from the antiperspirant and put in a cold place for complete solidification.

After a couple of days, the deodorant will become harder.

Application: apply to the skin of the armpits with a thin layer without much effort. This will make your deodorant invisible on the skin and increase its lifespan. For sensitive skin, the amount of corn starch should be increased to 80 g, and soda should be reduced to 30 g.

It is recommended to store in the refrigerator. This deodorant can be prepared in two forms, solid and powdered. Powdered deodorant differs from solid in the absence of coconut oil. They need to gently slap the skin of the armpits.

One more popular thing is beeswax. It might become a good basis for your natural deodorant. Thus, the next recipe is **solid natural deodorant with beeswax**. To prepare it, take 6 grams of beeswax, 24 grams of coconut or palm oil, 24 grams of baking soda, 16 grams of corn or potato starch, and finally 15 drops of essential oils.

Go through this list step by step:

1. 1.Mix well soda and starch.

2. Melt beeswax in a water bath, send coconut oil or palm oil to be heated there.

3. Pour mixed soda with starch into the resulting substance and mix everything.

4. Add essential oils and mix everything thoroughly. Put the mixture in a silicone mold for ice or in a deodorant tube. Put in the fridge until it solidifies.

Due to the presence of beeswax, such a deodorant in the refrigerator is not necessary to store. Essential oils for natural home deodorants can be chosen in accordance to your preferences. Otherwise, you might listen to the advice of those who are experts.

For example, you have a wide range to choose from, especially, tea tree, lavender, verbena, rosewood, vanilla, geranium, juniper, nutmeg, pine, spruce, palmarosa, and vetiver.

However, once you can boast sensitive skin, you need something different. Well, thank to a huge variety of natural materials, there is nothing easier than choosing the one you need for your skin.

Natural deodorant for sensitive skin is going to be prepared like that. You have to take one tablespoon of corn or potato starch . one tablespoon of baking soda, one tablespoon of beeswas, the same amount of coconut or cedar oil, pour refined shea butter (as well, 1 tsp), add stearic acid at the tip of a knife and put from three to five drops of essential oils.

After the fundamental is ready, do the following actions:

1. Mix soda and starch together.
2. On a water bath, melt the wax, shea butter, coconut oil (cedar)
3. Mix the mixture with soda and starch.

4. Add stearic acid and essential oils.
5. Mix everything thoroughly. Transfer to a container from a deodorant or in a mold.
6. Leave in the refrigerator until full freezing.

Chapter 5 – The best ways to use aloe in natural deodorants

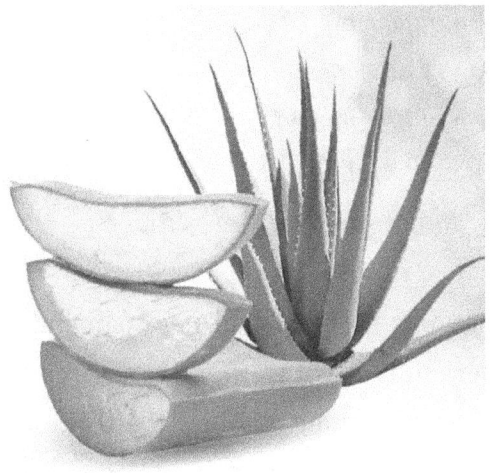

The natural deodorants are based on natural absorbents that take away sweat and odor neutralizing agents. Usually it is clay, soda, essential oils. You can also choose the form of a deodorant, particularly, opt for liquid or solid one. The second most popular component after the coconut is aloe. Especially, it is indispensable once you have decided to **make a solid deodorant**.

To prepare your own smell, you don't need to get a special education of perfumer. Instead, take the following ingredients:

1/4 cup coconut oil

1/4 cup shea butter,

1/4 cup beeswax granules

1 tablespoon glycerin,

1 tablespoon of aloe vera gel,

1 tablespoon of baking soda,

20 drops of essential oil of tea tree or eucalyptus,

20 drops of mint or lavender essential oil.

Melt the beeswax oil in a small saucepan and add glycerin and aloe vera to it. Mix the oil mixture, soda and essential oils in a separate container. Allow the mixture to cool and pour into old deodorant packaging. You can also pour the mixture into silicone molds for cupcakes.

As we have already discussed the importance of natural deodorants, it might look like a spray. If you are into such kinds of things, study the benefits of the natural components.

To make **spray deodorant at home**, take one spray bottle, 1/4 cup of strong alcohol, vinegar (actually, it might be unfiltered apple, but you can also use plain white) - 2 teaspoons. Next, don't forget about a pinch of natural salt (as well, it is good idea to choose pink Himalayan or sea one).

As well, why don't you take essential oils? Their amount may vary to your taste (for example, you are likely to get a good smell having combined lavender and geranium oil). Generally, it is advised to take 15 drops of each essential oil. Additionally, take one tablespoon of aloe.

The method of preparation includes the following steps:

1. 1)Pour salt in a bottle, add essential oils, aloe vera and pour alcohol and a bite.

2. 2) Shake well. Thus, you have seen how easy it is to prepare it at home. Once we have talked about the usage, after a shower or bath, sprinkle 2-3 times in the right place.

Actually, while making a choice in favor of natural aloe deodorant, you should consider some important facts:

- Give your armpits time to get used to the natural deodorant. The first days of use you probably have to put more. But over time, the glands will change and you will sweat less and the unpleasant smell will disappear.

- When applied to freshly shaved skin, it will pinch!

- Deodorant will not smell of vinegar, but only the essential oils that you add to them. So feel free to combine your favorite smells!

- Using this deodorant you will sweat! What you should do! Sweating is a way to remove toxins from our body, so in no case should we stop it.

- This deodorant does not whiten and does not leave stains on clothes.

As there are a lot of recipes of spray deodorants which you might prepare at home, you can **try another option**. Spray differs in an economic expense, as well, it can be taken with itself in the road.

1. Fill with cold water (250 ml) a couple of tablespoons of dry herbal. Pharmacy chamomile, train, linden have excellent antibacterial action.

2. Bring the infusion to a boil, hold on the fire for 15-20 minutes, cool and strain.

3. Add 2-4 tbsp. tablespoons of baking soda and the same amount of aloe juice.

4. The role of fragrance performs any essential oil - 6-7 drops is enough.

5. Stir the mixture thoroughly, pour into a bottle with a spray. Store in a dry cool place for no more than a week. Before use, be sure to shake the bottle so that there is no sediment.

To make a liquid deodorant at home, mix baking soda and cornstarch and add a few drops of your favorite essential oil, such as lavender. Natural liquid deodorants can also be prepared by mixing the extract of witch hazel, aloe vera juice, mineral water, glycerin and antibacterial essential oils.

Alum has been used for personal hygiene for many centuries. Mineral crystals are also used as natural deodorants, since they create an environment in which bacteria cannot multiply. Mineral crystals kill bacteria that cause an unpleasant odor.

Chapter 6 – For those who love fruits: how to combine citrus with grapefruit in your deodorant

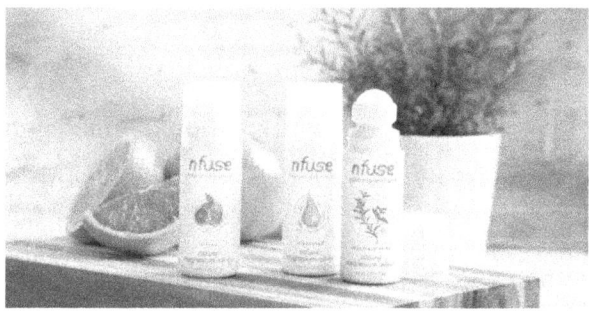

Liquid natural deodorant at home is the easiest to prepare. It consists almost entirely of vegetable oils, which are strictly metered and selected in such a way as not to leave greasy marks on clothes.

To make a liquid deodorant at home with your own hands, you will need 5 milliliters of grape seed oil (as well, you might use sesame instead), 7-10 drops of tea tree oil, 5 drops of rosemary oil (you can substitute geranium oil or palmarosa), 15 drops of lavender oil, and bottle deodorant roller

Grape seed oil contributes to the rapid absorption and drying of funds, tea tree gives an excellent antiseptic, and various essential oils are added to bring a pleasant aroma to the composition.

All components after adding to the bottle should be thoroughly shaken. If it is not possible to add all the listed oils, then you can use only the required - grape seed oil, tea tree and rosemary.

In the warm season, try not to use deodorant orange, lemon and grapefruit oil for making your own hands. They are very susceptible to the heat of the sun and if you go to sunbathe using this tool, you run the risk of severe burns.

Inflicting deodorant, it should be allowed to soak. This will happen within 5-7 minutes. You can store it for 3 weeks in a dry dark place. Such a deodorant, cooked with your own hands, does not leave marks on clothes and perfectly eliminates unpleasant odor. If you feel that the aroma has evaporated, you can safely add a few drops of a little heated essential oil to the composition.

It is believed it that the following citrus recipe for **homemade deodorant** originates in ancient Egypt, and it was used by verily famous Queen Cleopatra. Take the juice of your favorite citrus and mix it with a small amount of cinnamon. Pay attention that as a result of mixing you should get a mixture that has the consistency, like sour cream.

As well, you might add in the following substance some rose oil that should be applied in a small amount. As a deodorant, such a combination which included rose oil it was first used in India. To make the effect better, before applying, mix rose oil with any base oil (olive, peach and so on): for one tablespoon of base oil, 6 drops of rose oil.

Citrus homemade deodorant will be perfect for everyone who loves the fresh aroma of oranges and lemons. For its manufacture will need 0.5 tablespoons of beeswax, 2 tablespoons of coconut oil, 2 tablespoons of baking soda, 1 tablespoon of corn starch, 10-15 drops of essential oil (you can use several flavors at once). Beeswax must be melted, then mix coconut oil with it. Soda and cornstarch should be poured into the resulting billet, mix thoroughly and add essential oils.

The mixture is placed in a tube and put to cool. Take your time using the deodorant you made. The finished mixture takes time to harden. As a rule, it is enough for this from several hours to one day.

Apply a deodorant in a very thin layer, without pressure. If you did everything correctly, no trace of the product on the skin (and even more so on clothing) should remain.

Chapter 7 – Rose deodorants: when fragrance is the most important

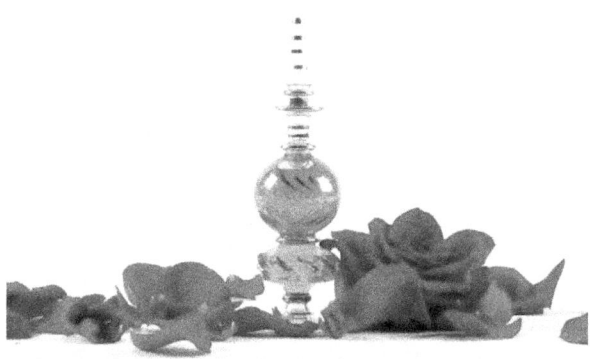

The deodorants with the rose components are usually based on the structure which you have already studied very well from the previous recipes. You might take the basis and add rose oil in such an amount which seems great for you. For example, let's look at the following recipe of **rose deodorant**.

Firstly, take 25 g of soda,15 g of corn starch, 30 g coconut oil, and rose oil. At the beginning, mix the right amount of soda with starch. Soda has long been considered the best way to combat the smell of sweat, because it creates an alkaline environment that destroys bacteria.

Starch absorbs moisture quickly, so the armpits will always be dry. Add coconut oil. It melts at 24 degrees, so when applied to the skin, the deodorant will melt slightly and slide well. You can also add a couple of drops of your favorite rose essential oil. Just remember that you will feel this smell all day, so choose a pleasant scent for yourself.

Place the resulting mass in a deodorant box, tamp well. This tool should be stored in the refrigerator. Self-made deodorant is harmless and does not violate the natural processes in the body. Of course, you need to get used to it, but the result will pleasantly surprise you. With proper use, such a deodorant is very economical, and you can check its effectiveness right now!

Liquid deodorant with alum also might contain the component of rose. It will bring you unforgettable fragrance. As well, it is hard while preparing. To make it, take 5 gr of aluminum alum, 40 gr of distilled water, Vitamin E, and 5 gr of Glycerin.

Additional ingredients are the following ones:
- *Shea butter - 5 gr.*
- *Rosemary hydrolat (deodorant itself) - 15 ml.*

- *Rose hydrolat (antibacterial properties) - 15 ml.*
- *Xanthan or guar (gelling agent) - 1 gr.*
- *Malavit (has healing and deodorizing qualities) - 30 cap.*
- *Aloe, liquid extract or aloe juice (moisturizes, relieves irritation) - 6 ml.*
- *Chlorophyllite alcohol (preservative) - 1 tsp.*
- *Essential oils are necessary, so jasmine and orange are well combined.*

To prepare it, do the following things:

1. Pour distilled water into a container, pour alum, put in a bath 40 degrees, stir until alum is dissolved.

2. Pour herbal distillate, xanthan or guar. At this stage, the water should be warm enough, but not boiling water, so that the hydrolates would not lose their properties. Mix well to dissolve the gel.

3. Add the remaining ingredients.

4. Beat with a blender or mixer, or just a fork.

5. Wash the bottle and roller of industrial deodorant, dry, spray it with alcohol to disinfect and pour deodorant.

Alum significantly reduces the secretion of sebaceous and sweat glands, is a strong antiperspirant, and has a deodorizing effect. Unlike aluminum, which is commonly used in industrial deodorants, which penetrates the blood and accumulates in the internal organs, forms plugs in the sweat glands, potassium alum does not penetrate into the cells and do not disrupt the work of the sweat glands.

Their action is based on high adsorption properties. Alum destroy bacterial cells, whose vital activity is the source of the smell. This deodorant absorbs quickly and pleasantly lubricates and moisturizes.

Conclusion

If you love natural cosmetics and products for the care of natural ingredients, you must have thought about changing your deodorant. Unfortunately, most of the deodorants that we see on the shelves of supermarkets are unsafe and often contain harmful substances.

And although we are accustomed to first of all pay attention to the duration of the protection effect and a pleasant smell - this is not at all the most important thing. That composition should be the main argument to buy or not to buy a product.

How to choose a deodorant? Give preference to products that consist solely of natural ingredients. They destroy the germs that cause unpleasant odor, capable of essential oils. In natural deodorants which, by the way, you can prepare on your own there are potassium alum, soda, zinc oxide, starch and extracts of medicinal herbs.

These components are not toxic, but they will save you from an unpleasant smell not worse than ordinary deodorants. So, find your best recipe and make a unique product!

www.ingramcontent.com/pod-product-compliance
Lightning Source LLC
Chambersburg PA
CBHW070453290526
45791CB00005B/2122